Focuse
MRCS Finals (OSCE)

J Kean

C Stephen

J Hughes

S Enoch

Foreword by

Professor R J C Steele

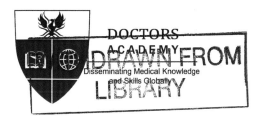

1st Edition, May 2010, Doctors Academy Publications

Focused Clinical Examination for MRCS Finals (OSCE)

Authors

Ms Jennifer Kean, BMSc (Hons), MBChB, MRCSEd
Duke of Kent Plastic Surgery Research Fellow
Stoke Mandeville Hospital, Buckinghamshire

Mr Chris Stephen, MBChB, MRCS
Speciality Trainee in Plastic Surgery
University Hospital of Central Manchester

Ms Juliana M F Hughes, BSc (Hons), MBChB, MRCS(Ed)
Speciality Registrar in Plastic Surgery
South-West Deanery
Frenchay Hospital, Bristol

Mr Stuart Enoch, MBBS, MRCSEd, MRCS (Eng), PhD
Speciality Registrar in Plastic Surgery
North West Deanery
Manchester, United Kingdom

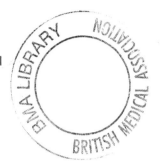

Foreword by

Professor R J C Steele
BSc, MB ChB, MD, FRCS Ed, FRCS Eng (Ad Eundum), FCS (HK)
Professor of Surgery and Head of Academic Surgery
Centre for Academic Clinical Practice
Ninewells Hospital & Medical School, Dundee, UK

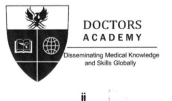

DOCTORS
ACADEMY
Disseminating Medical Knowledge
and Skills Globally

ALL RIGHTS RESERVED

1st Edition, May 2010, Doctors Academy Publications

Electronic version published at	:	Doctors Academy, PO Box 4283 Cardiff,CF14 8GN,United Kingdom
Print version printed and published at	:	Abbey Bookbinding and Print Co., Unit 3, Gabalfa Workshops, Clos Menter, Cardiff CF14 3AY
ISBN	:	978-93-80573-14-4
Cover page Design	:	Sreekanth S.S
Type Setting	:	Lakshmi Sreekanth
Contact	:	publishing@doctorsacademy.org.uk

Preface

A meticulous yet concise clinical examination forms the cornerstone of surgical practice. With the introduction of the new MRCS OSCE style examination, clinical skills are now tested alongside core knowledge and fundamental surgical principles, and its application in everyday practice. Whereas previous MRCS candidates had valuable study time between passing the viva and sitting the clinical exam, candidates appearing from the OSCE style must simultaneously balance knowledge-based study with their clinical examination skills.

This book provides a focused approach to the individual clinical examination stations and highlights essential aspects that the candidate should cover in each station to accrue sufficient marks to pass the clinical examination skills component of the OSCE. In addition, the types of clinical scenarios and some of the commonly asked questions in the various stations are also highlighted. Whilst more detailed texts exist to introduce students to the nuances and complexities of clinical examination, the authors intend this book to be used for simple and accessible revision of the skills necessary to succeed in the modern MRCS OSCE.

Good luck with your exam preparation!

- JK
- CS
- JH
- SE

Foreword

The MRCS OSCE focuses on clinical skills and a successful candidate has to demonstrate a logical and precise approach to clinical examination. The structure of the exam, however, is such that individual components of clinical examination are tested rather than taking a global approach. Thus, this book on Focused Clinical Examination is highly relevant for trainees preparing for the final MRCS. It must be borne in mind, however, that the MRCS examination is not an end in itself but rather a beginning. As you progress through higher surgical training, the importance of clinical examination does not diminish and this book will act as a vade mecum well beyond the period of preparation for the exam. It is clear, practical and beautifully produced. I wish it and its authors well.

Professor R J C Steele,
BSc, MB ChB, MD, FRCS Ed, FRCS Eng (Ad Eundum), FCS (HK)
Professor of Surgery and Head of Academic Surgery
Centre for Academic Clinical Practice
Ninewells Hospital & Medical School, Dundee, UK

Acknowledgements

The authors wish to thank Mr Mathew Briggs of the Medical Illustration Department, Royal Preston Hospital, for his patience and skill in obtaining all photographs for this book. Further thanks to Miss Joanne Green for being such an excellent simulated-patient and model.

Contents

CHAPTER 1

ABDOMEN

POSSIBLE QUESTIONS YOU MAY GET ASKED:

- Examine this patient's abdomen
- Examine the liver / spleen / kidneys / scrotum / groin
- Examine this patient with jaundice
- Examine this patient for signs of liver disease / inflammatory bowel disease / colonic cancer
- Examine this patient's hernia
- Examine this patient's stoma

1. Introduce yourself and ask permission to examine

2. Position and Exposure

Position the patient flat on the couch and expose the abdomen, preserving the patient's dignity by keeping the groin covered unless exposure is needed.

3. General Inspection from end of bed

- Does the patient look comfortable?
- How is the general appearance and nutritional status?
- Is there any obvious pallor or jaundice?
- Are there drains, stomas etc

4. Perform a general examination of the patient

The examiners may tell you to skip this step, move on or specify that you examine only the abdomen.

THE HANDS

Nails

- Anaemia
- Clubbing (Crohn's disease, Ulcerative colitis, Cirrhosis)

- Leuconychia (Caused by hypoproteinaemia associated with liver disease)
- **Koilonychia (Spoon shaped nails seen in iron deficiency anaemia)**

Check for **Asterixis** (liver flap), seen in decompensated liver disease

THE FACE

Eyes

- Anaemia (pale conjunctiva)
- Jaundice

Mouth

- Dentition
- Ulcers (Inflammatory bowel disease, herpes simplex)
- Tongue
    ‣ Dehydration
    ‣ Smooth, red, beefy (B12 deficiency)
- Angular stomatitis
    ‣ Caused by iron, folate and vitamin B/C deficiency
    ‣ Also seen in herpes simplex and oral candidiasis
- Hepatic Foetor

Spider naevi can be seen in the face.

THE ARMS & TRUNK

- Spider Naevi are found along the distribution of the Superior Vena Cava (i.e., above the nipple line) and are associated with oestrogen excess
    ‣ More than five are significant in women
    ‣ The presence of any is significant in men
- Purpura, petechiae
    ‣ Can be caused by low platelets or raised prothrombin time
- Gynaecomastia
- Signs of pruritus – scratch marks

SUPRACLAVICULAR LYMPH NODES

Virchow's Node in the left supraclavicular fossa can be enlarged in gastric cancer.

Kean J, Stephen C, Hughes J, Enoch S. Focused Clinical Examination for
MRCS Finals (OSCE). Doctors Academy Publications

5. Examine the abdomen

a) Inspect **for**

- Scratch marks
- Swelling, distension
- Caput medusae
- Skin changes (bruising, signs of weight loss)
- Scars
- Striae
- Any visible pulsations

Ask the patient to cough or lift his/her head off the bed to reveal any herniae or signs of peritonism (unlikely in the exam!). Do not forget to do this as this can reveal considerable pathology and allow you to focus the rest of the examination.

b) Palpate

Important points before starting:
- Kneel down at the patient's right side
- Ask the patient if there is any generalised pain or localised pain
- Palpate all nine distinct areas of the abdomen starting furthest from you, unless the patient indicates an area of pain, in which case palpate this area last
- Look at patient's face for signs of pain while palpating
- Palpate the abdomen with flattened fingers (**Figure 1.1**)

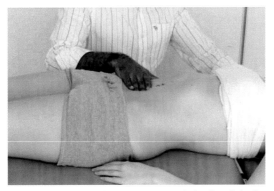

Figure 1.1: Palpation of the abdomen with the flat of the fingers

Kean J, Stephen C, Hughes J, Enoch S. Focused Clinical Examination for MRCS Finals (OSCE). Doctors Academy Publications

Deep palpation for masses (liver, spleen, kidneys)
Now palpate all nine areas deeply, feeling for masses.

Liver:

• Start in the right iliac fossa, asking the patient to take deep breaths in and out. Move your hand upwards towards the costal margin during inspiration until you feel a liver edge on expiration (**Figure 1.2**).

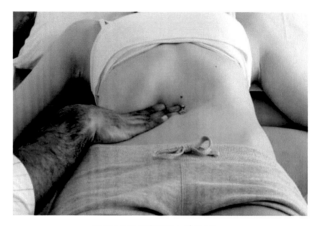

Figure 1.2: Palpation of the liver

• If the liver is palpable check the
  ▸ Size (record enlargement in cm below costal margin)
  ▸ Texture (soft / firm / hard / nodular)
  ▸ Edge (smooth / irregular)
    ▪ An irregular liver edge suggests metastases

Superficial palpation, checking for

• Tenderness
• Rigidity
• Guarding

Kean J, Stephen C, Hughes J, Enoch S. Focused Clinical Examination for
MRCS Finals (OSCE). Doctors Academy Publications

Gallbladder:

Feel under the liver edge for a palpable gallbladder (**Figure 1.3**).

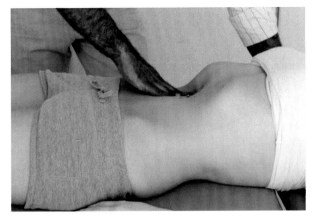

Figure 1.3: Palpation of the gallbladder

Murphy's test: With your hand in the position of the gallbladder, fingers pointing up, ask the patient to take a deep breath in and out. Pain on expiration as the gallbladder comes to rest against your fingertips is a positive Murphy's test.

Spleen:

Start palpating in the right iliac fossa, using the same breathing technique as for liver palpation. However, this time move gradually towards the left upper quadrant (**Figure 1.4**). Note the size, texture and edge of the spleen.

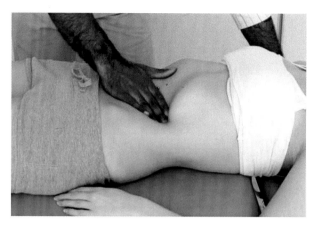

Figure 1.4: Palpation of the spleen

Kidneys:

'Ballot' the kidneys using both hands (**Figure 1.5**).

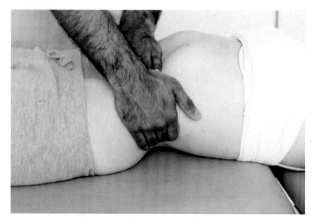

Figure 1.5: 'Balloting' the kidneys

Abdominal aorta:

Palpate in the region of the lower epigastrium/upper umbilical area, slightly towards the left of the mid-line, deeply for a pulsatile mass. Note the approximate diameter by using both hands to feel the lateral edges of the mass. *(Note that the abdominal aorta may be easily palpable in patients with minimal abdominal fat/thin abdominal musculature).*

c) Percuss **for**

• Upper liver border (**Figure 1.6**)

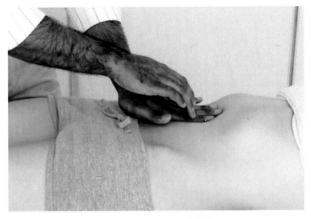

Figure 1.6: Percussion of the liver

• Spleen
• Bladder (**Figure 1.7**)

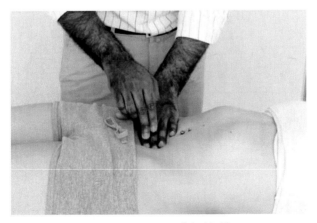

Figure 1.7: Percussion of the bladder

Kean J, Stephen C, Hughes J, Enoch S. Focused Clinical Examination for MRCS Finals (OSCE). Doctors Academy Publications

- Ascites: Start by percussing in the midline towards either flank and note any change in pitch from resonant to dull, indicating fluid (**Figure 1.8**). If there is dullness, keep your finger on this area and ask the patient to roll onto his/her side so that the dull area is now superior.

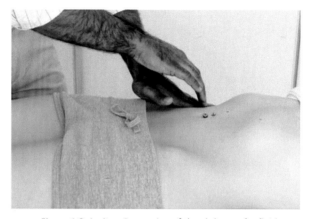

Figure 1.8: Ascites: Percussion of the abdomen for fluid

Percuss again and note any change in pitch back to resonance (**Figure 1.9**). If present, this is shifting dullness.

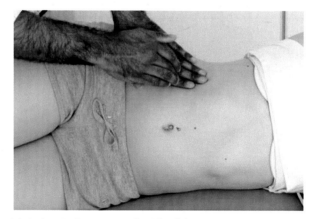

Figure 1.9: Ascites: Patient turns to the side whilst percussion position is maintained; listen for altered percussion note

Kean J, Stephen C, Hughes J, Enoch S. Focused Clinical Examination for MRCS Finals (OSCE). Doctors Academy Publications

d) Auscultate

- Over the left iliac fossa for bowel sounds
- Over the liver for a bruit
- Over the aorta, iliac vessels and the renal arteries for bruits

If you have not yet found any abnormality, tell the examiner you would like to expose the genitalia and examine the groin, inguinal canal and femoral pulses.

6. Examination of male genitalia

Listen clearly to the examiner's instruction, which will usually indicate if the problem is in the groin or scrotum. If instructed to examine the groin, begin by examining for inguinal herniae before moving onto the scrotum.

a) Position & exposure

The patient may be supine, sitting or standing. If supine, remember to ask him to stand at the end so that a varicocoele is not missed. If sitting in a chair or standing, then request the patient to stand up and examine him standing. Ensure adequate exposure of the groin and scrotum.

b) Inspection

- Inspect the groin and scrotum looking for any obvious swellings
- Ask the patient to cough
- Look for surgical scars in the groin (may have been used for testicular approach) and scrotum (may be difficult to see as they are often in the median raphe)

c) Palpation

- Remember to enquire about pain first
- Place the fingers of one hand behind the testis and palpate using the other (**Figure 1.10**). Use the thumb to assess the normal contour. The surface should be smooth and regular.

Kean J, Stephen C, Hughes J, Enoch S. Focused Clinical Examination for MRCS Finals (OSCE). Doctors Academy Publications

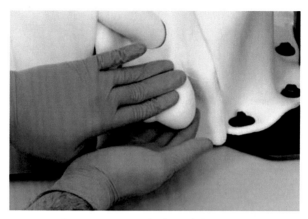

Figure 1.10: Bimanual palpation of the testicle

- Identify the epididymis and vas deferens
- Palpate the spermatic cord between thumb and index finger (**Figure 1.11**)

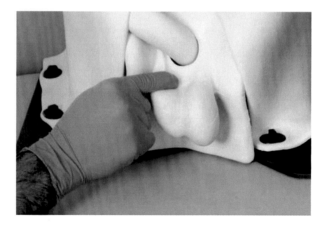

Figure 1.1: Palpation of the spermatic cord between the thumb and index finger

- If there is a lump :
  - ▸ Is it separate from the testis?
  - ▸ Does it transilluminate?
  - ▸ Can you get above it?

Kean J, Stephen C, Hughes J, Enoch S. Focused Clinical Examination for MRCS Finals (OSCE). Doctors Academy Publications

Complete the examination by saying you would like to examine the rest of the groin and abdomen if you have not done so already. Remember that the lymphatic drainage of the testes is to the para-aortic nodes, which will not be palpable. The penis and scrotal skin, however, drains to the inguinal nodes, so if there is pathology here (i.e., Squamous Cell Carcinoma) you should examine the inguinal nodes.

7. Special examinations

A) TESTICULAR TUMOURS

It is uncommon to have these patients in the exam but you should be prepared to describe the clinical features that would make you suspect a testicular tumour:

- A hard, irregular, 'craggy' mass
- Inseparable from the testis
- Non-tender
- Non trans-illuminable
- You can get above it
- Tell the examiner that you would complete the examination by palpating for hepatomegaly and listening to the chest (for liver and lung metastases)

B) HERNIAE

You should approach hernia examination in the same manner as you would for abdominal examination, starting with the hands. The examiner, however, will often move you straight to the hernia examination.

Inguinal Hernia

This is a very common case and you should be comfortable examining inguinal herniae. Be prepared to explain as you define the anatomy and present your findings clearly – although relatively straightforward, candidates often get it wrong, losing easy marks. The patient is likely to be supine - if you cannot detect the lump on this position ask the patient to stand. Otherwise it is not necessary to examine in both lying and standing positions.

Inspection

- Scars (this may be a recurrent hernia or they may have had a previous hernia on the contralateral side)
- If the swelling is not obvious ask the patient to cough or lift his/her head off the bed
- If you still cannot see a hernia, ask the patient if he/she has noticed any lumps in their groin
- Describe what you see (as for any lump).

Palpation

- If the hernia is not reduced when you commence your examination, ask the patient if he/she can reduce it themselves. If not, gently reduce the hernia, making sure you enquire about pain and observe the patient's face
- Take your time to define the anatomy, identifying the pubic tubercle and anterior superior iliac spine. The inguinal ligament runs in between these points and the deep inguinal ring is just above its' mid-point (this is the mid-point of the inguinal ligament). If the pubic tubercle is not easily defined, palpate the adductor longus muscle by flexing, abducting and externally rotating the thigh – the pubic tubercle is its point of insertion.
- Feel for a cough impulse (ask the patient to cough)
- Examine as you would for any lump (consistency, reducibility etc)
- Does the lump extend into the scrotum?
- With the hernia reduced, redefine the anatomy, place two fingers over the deep ring and ask the patient to cough. If the hernia is controlled at the deep ring, it is said to be INDIRECT. If it is not controlled it will usually come out medial to the deep ring and is said to be DIRECT.
- Remember that this is an inaccurate test, with inaccuracy reported to be up to 50%. However, it is a good way to test knowledge of the inguinal canal and you will be expected to differentiate clinically between direct and indirect herniae.
- Complete the examination by asking to examine the scrotum and contralateral groin.

Kean J, Stephen C, Hughes J, Enoch S. Focused Clinical Examination for MRCS Finals (OSCE). Doctors Academy Publications

Femoral Hernia

You are very unlikely to encounter a femoral hernia in the exam as they usually present acutely and, as such, frequently require prompt surgical intervention. You will, however, be expected to know the difference between a femoral and inguinal hernia clinically, as well as the differential diagnosis of a lump in the groin.

In femoral hernia:

• The hernia arises below the inguinal ligament
• They are twice as common in females than males
• The risk of strangulation is high
• Cough impulse is usually absent
• They are usually irreducible

Other herniae

The examinations for incisional, umbilical and epigastric herniae are essentially the same, so we will consider these together. With an incisional hernia, the patient will have an abdominal scar (often large). As this is a short case, there can be more than one problem to identify in this station so be prepared to move on after you have identified the hernia.

Inspection

• Describe any scars and look for other scars, stomas etc
• Ask the patient to lift their head off the bed and look for bulging of the hernia or scar

Palpation

• Enquire about tenderness and palpate the hernia, commenting on any defect you can feel
• Ask the patient to cough and demonstrate weakness in the scar or abdominal wall, feeling for bulging of abdominal contents against your hand
• Try to determine the size of the defect
• If there is a midline longitudinal abdominal bulging with no scar, consider divarication of the recti.

Kean J, Stephen C, Hughes J, Enoch S. Focused Clinical Examination for MRCS Finals (OSCE). Doctors Academy Publications

Auscultate

• Listen for bowel sounds

Completion

• Tell the examiner that you would move on to examine the rest of the abdomen if you have not already done so.

C) STOMAS

If you are asked to examine a patient with a stoma you will usually be instructed to inspect only. Do not touch the patient unless you are instructed to. You should be familiar with the different types of stoma and their relevant sites. If there is a bag covering the stoma you may only be expected to comment on the site and contents before moving onto the rest of the abdomen.

Inspection

• Site
• Mucosal lining
• Is there a spout or is it flush with the skin?
• Number of openings – end (1) vs. loop (2)
• Contents of the bag (colour, consistency)
• Do not get confused by a urostomy or cholecystostomy
• Inspect the rest of the abdomen (scars, other stomas or previous stoma sites)

8. To complete the examination of the abdomen

Say you would like to

• Feel the hernial orifices
• Examine external genitalia (e.g., for testicular atrophy in chronic liver disease)
• Perform a rectal examination
• Examine the lower limbs for peripheral oedema
• Carry out a urine dipstick

9. Thank the patient

BE PREPARED TO ANSWER QUESTIONS ON:

Jaundice

- How can jaundice be classified and what are the major causes?
- How would you investigate a patient with surgical jaundice?
- Please interpret these liver function tests!

Hepatomegaly

- How would you investigate a patient with hepatomegaly?
- What are the causes of hepatomegaly?
- What is portal hypertension?

Splenomegaly

- What are the functions of the spleen?
- What are the causes of splenomegaly?
- What are the causes of massive splenomegaly?
- What are the indications for a splenectomy?
- How would you perform a splenectomy?
- What immunizations are required post-splenectomy?

Transplanted Kidney

- *Clinical signs may include:*

  ▶ a scar from an AV fistula present at the wrist
  ▶ signs of anaemia and steroid use
  ▶ a swelling in the right or left iliac fossa with an overlying curved scar from a Rutherford-Morrison incision
  ▶ previous nephrectomy scars
  ▶ a superficial and well defined mass, requiring only light palpation to identify

- *Questions:*

  ▶ What are the indications for renal transplantation?
  ▶ What occurs in transplant rejection and how would you identify it?
  ▶ What is the blood supply of a transplanted kidney?

Kean J, Stephen C, Hughes J, Enoch S. Focused Clinical Examination for MRCS Finals (OSCE). Doctors Academy Publications

Enlarged Kidney

An enlarged kidney will descend with inspiration, may be palpated bimanually and will be resonant to percussion because of overlying bowel. The examining hand can get in between the swelling and the costal margin.

• What are the causes of an enlarged kidney?
• What is the normal presentation of renal cell carcinoma?
• What are the differences between infantile and adult polycystic kidney disease?

Ascites

• What are the causes of ascites?
• In which conditions would you expect a transudate / exudate?
• How can ascites be managed?

Hydrocoele

• *Clinical signs may include:*

  ‣ a firm swelling
  ‣ inseparable from the testis (unless it is a hydrocoele of the cord)
  ‣ transillumination
  ‣ The examining fingers can get above it.

• *Questions:*

  ‣ What is a hydrocoele?
  ‣ What are the treatment options (surgical & non-surgical)?
  ‣ What is the anatomical classification of hydrocoeles?

Varicocele

• *Clinical signs may include:*

  ‣ The affected testis may hang lower on inspection.
  ‣ Varicoceles won't usually appear unless the patient is standing up.
  ‣ There is a swelling which:

- Is separate from the testis
- Is non-transilluminable
- Feels like a 'bag of worms'
- You can get above and may have a palpable cough impulse

- *Questions:*

  - What is a varicocele?
  - Give reasons (about three) why 98% of varicoceles are left-sided?
  - What are the treatment options?

Epididymal Cyst:

- *Clinical signs may include:*

  - The scrotum will usually appear normal on inspection.
  - There is a firm swelling within the epididymis, separate from the testis.
  - May transilluminate unless it contains sperm.
  - You can get above the mass.

- *Questions:*

  - What causes epididymal cysts?
  - What are the treatment options?

Testicular Tumours

- Describe the differential diagnosis (scarring from chronic infection, a long-standing hydrocoele with calcification)
- How do these tumours present?
- Describe the differences between teratomas and seminomas
- How is a testicular tumour removed?

Inguinal Hernia

- Describe the anatomy of the inguinal canal
- What is the difference between a direct and indirect hernia?
- What are the contents of the spermatic cord? (three arteries, three nerves, three other structures...)

- How would you perform a hernia repair?
- What are the potential complications?
- What would you tell the patient about recovery from a hernia repair?

When explaining treatment options for hernia, ensure that you consider non-surgical and surgical treatments. Remember to mention that you would address and control anaesthetic risk factors prior to surgery, particularly cardio-respiratory disease, as well as encouraging weight-loss.

Incisional Hernia

- What is an incisional hernia?
- What are the predisposing factors?
- What are the complications of incisional hernia?
- What are the treatment options?

Umbilical Hernia

- What is the pathogenesis of umbilical hernia?
- Do they require surgical repair in both adults and children? In children they usually resolve spontaneously but repair is advised in adults, as the risk of strangulation is high.
- How would you repair an umbilical hernia?

Epigastric Hernia

- What is an epigastric hernia and how do they commonly present?
- What are the treatment options?

Stomas

- What are the indications for a stoma?
- How can you tell the difference between an ileostomy and a colostomy?
- How would you prepare a patient preoperatively for a stoma?
- What are the (specific and general) complications of a stoma?

CHAPTER 2

BACK

1. Introduce yourself and ask permission to examine

2. Inspect with patient standing

From behind look for

• Muscle wasting
• Asymmetry
• Scoliosis
• Swellings
• Scars
• Abnormal skin creases, hair distribution or pigmentation (these can indicate Spina Bifida)

From the side look for

• Loss of lumbar or cervical lordosis
• Exaggerated thoracic kyphosis or cervical lordosis

From the front look for

• Alignment of the pelvis
• Chest wall deformities

If there is a scoliosis ask the patient to

▸ Sit down to exclude a compensatory scoliosis (in leg length discrepancy)
▸ Bend forward to exclude a postural scoliosis (which occurs most commonly in adolescent girls and usually resolves spontaneously)

Only then can a structural scoliosis be diagnosed.

3. Feel

Ask the patient whether there is any localised pain

▸ Feel down spinous processes and over sacroiliac joints, examining for steps or obvious tenderness

- Palpate paraspinal muscles for tenderness.
- Lightly percuss from neck to sacroiliac joints with the ulnar border of your fist (**Figure 2.1**).

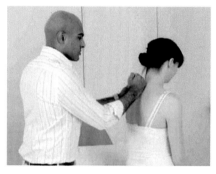

Figure 2.1: Light percussion from neck to sacroiliac joints with the ulnar border of fist

4. Move

With patient standing, examine lumbar and thoracic spine

- Check for chest expansion (**Figure 2.2**). This should be at least 5cm.

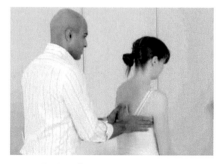

Figure 2.2: Checking for chest expansion (should be at least 5cm)

Kean J, Stephen C, Hughes J, Enoch S. Focused Clinical Examination for MRCS Finals (OSCE). Doctors Academy Publications

▸ Flexion and Schrober's test

▸ Extension

▸ Lateral flexion

▸ Rotation (ask the patient to cross his/xher arms across his/her chest and either fix the pelvis with your hands on the patient's hips, or ask him/her to sit)

Schrober's test: Mark a point midline between the dimples of Venus and another point 10cm above it (**Figure 2.3**).

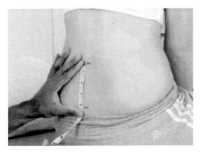

Figure 2.3: Schrober's test: Marks 10cm apart

The increase in distance between both points should be 8-10cm with flexion of the spine (bending forward) (**Figures 2.4 and 2.5**). Gross restriction (<3cm) can be seen in ankylosing spondylitis.

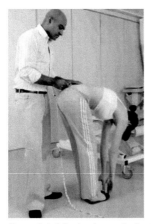

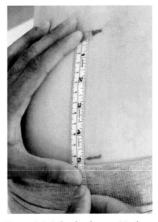

Figure 2.4: Schrober's test: Patient flexes the spine (bends forward)

Figure 2.5: Schrober's test: Marks now 12.5cm apart

Kean J, Stephen C, Hughes J, Enoch S. Focused Clinical Examination for MRCS Finals (OSCE). Doctors Academy Publications

With patient sitting, examine the cervical spine

▸ Flexion
▸ Extension
  • Feel for crepitations in flexion and extension, asking the patient to 'slowly nod' (often found in cervical osteoarthritis)
▸ Lateral flexion
▸ Rotation

5. Special tests

With patient supine

▸ Straight leg raise whilst the ankle is held in dorsiflexion (**Figure 2.6**)

  • Pain in thigh, buttock and back suggests sciatica (positive at L4 or below)

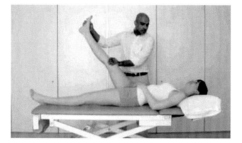

Figure 2.6: Straight leg raise with the ankle held in dorsiflexion

▸ Lasegue's test: foot neutral, knee flexed (**Figure 2.7**)

  • Hip can be flexed further without pain, but the pain reappears if the knee is then extended.

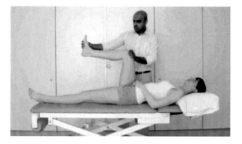

Figure 2.7 : Demonstration of Lasegue's test: Foot neutral, knee flexed

Kean J, Stephen C, Hughes J, Enoch S. Focused Clinical Examination for MRCS Finals (OSCE). Doctors Academy Publications

With patient prone

▸ Femoral nerve stretch test: extend the hip (**Figure 2.8**)

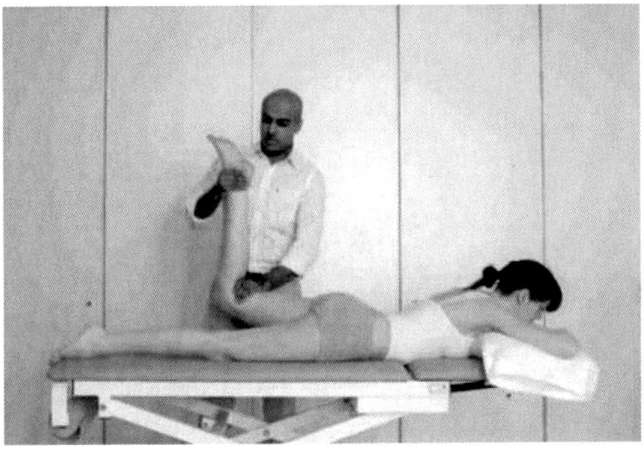

Figure 2.8 : Femoral nerve stretch test: Extending the hip

• Pain in thigh, buttock and back suggests nerve root irritation at L2-4

6. To complete the examination

Say you would also like to:

▸ Perform a neurological examination of upper and lower limbs

▸ Examine the abdomen (to exclude malignancy or aortic aneurysm as cause of back pain)

7. Thank the patient

Kean J, Stephen C, Hughes J, Enoch S. Focused Clinical Examination for MRCS Finals (OSCE). Doctors Academy Publications

BE PREPARED TO ANSWER QUESTIONS ON:

- Disc prolapse - tenderness over the lumbar spine is common in disc prolapse. Tenderness over lumbar muscles can be mechanical or secondary to disc prolapse
- Mechanical back pain
- Sciatica
- Spondylolisthesis - a step in the lumbar spine may be felt
- Ankylosing spondylitis – Most common in thoracic spine but can occur at other levels; has got a genetic predisposition.
- Metastatic deposits – e.g., Carcinoma of the Prostate can metastasise to the verbebrae

Kean J, Stephen C, Hughes J, Enoch S. Focused Clinical Examination for
MRCS Finals (OSCE). Doctors Academy Publications

CHAPTER 3

BREAST

POSSIBLE QUESTIONS YOU MAY GET ASKED:
- Examine this patient's breasts
- Examine for a breast lump

1. Introduce yourself and ask permission to examine

Remember the need for a chaperon!

2. Inspect the breasts with the patient uncovered above the waist

Position the patient sitting upright with hands on hips (**Figure 3.1**).
Look for

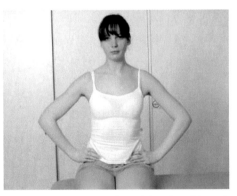

Figure 3.1: Position the patient sitting upright with hands on hips to inspect the breasts

- Breast symmetry
  - Size, shape, nipple position
- Nipple changes
  - Retraction, discharge, erosion
- Skin changes
  - Erythema, tethering, peau d'orange, lumps or lesions
  - Scars, radiotherapy tattoo or burns

- Changes in the arms or axillae
  ‣ Swelling, wasting, lymphoedema

Ask the patient to raise her arms and place them behind her head (**Figure 3.2**).

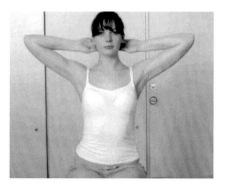

Figure 3.2: Position the patient sitting upright with hands behind head to inspect the breasts

Now look for asymmetry or tethering which may become apparent on changing position.

3. Feel

Ask about pain or tenderness before touching the patient. Ask if the patient has noticed any lumps; if so, examine the other breast first.
Position the patient lying reclined with a 45 degree tilt at the waist.
Use the flat of your fingers to palpate the breast (**Figure 3.3**)

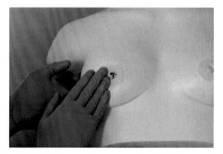

Figure 3.3: Use the flat of your fingers to palpate the breast in all four quadrants

Kean J, Stephen C, Hughes J, Enoch S. Focused Clinical Examination for MRCS Finals (OSCE). Doctors Academy Publications

- All four quadrants
- The central area and nipple areola complex
- The axillary tail.

Now examine the axilla

- Support the weight of the patient's arm with your arm – right for right or left for left
- Use your other hand to palpate the axilla – medial, posterior, anterior, lateral and the apex (**Figure 3.4** and **Figure 3.5**).

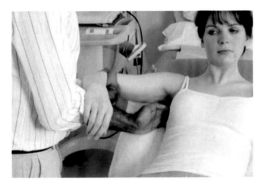

Figure 3.4: Palpation of the axilla: Medial and posterior group of lymph nodes

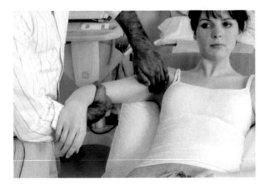

Figure 3.5: Palpation of the axilla: Anterior and lateral group of lymph nodes

Kean J, Stephen C, Hughes J, Enoch S. Focused Clinical Examination for MRCS Finals (OSCE). Doctors Academy Publications

Change sides and examine the other breast and axilla. If you find a lump, describe:

• Site
• Size
• Shape
• Skin surface
• Consistency
• Fluctuance
• Mobility or tethering – ask the patient to tense her chest muscles by pressing hands on hips whilst you attempt to move the lump parallel and perpendicular to the pectoralis major muscle fibres.

4. Special tests

• Examine for palpable lymph nodes in the supraclavicular fossae.

5. To complete the examination

Say you would also like to:

• Take a complete history of the lump including family history of breast disease
• Examine the abdomen and chest
• Plan for histopathology and imaging to complete triple assessment.

6. Ensure that they are re-dressed or covered

7. Thank the patient

BE PREPARED TO ANSWER QUESTIONS ON:

- Breast cysts
- Breast abscess and management
- Fibroadenoma – breast "mouse"
- Breast screening – Two-yearly mammography for ladies over the age of 50
- Triple assessment – Clinical exam, histopathology and imaging
- Breast cancer
- Axillary node sampling
- Axillary block dissection
- Sentinal node biopsy
- Mastectomy and options for reconstruction
- Lymphoedema post-axillary lymph node dissection and its management

Kean J, Stephen C, Hughes J, Enoch S. Focused Clinical Examination for
MRCS Finals (OSCE). Doctors Academy Publications

Exercise Page

CHAPTER 4

HAND

POSSIBLE QUESTIONS YOU MAY GET ASKED:

• Examine this patient's hands
• Assess this patient's joints
• Describe what you see in this patient's hands
• Assess this patient's neurological status of the upper limb
• Examine the median / ulnar / radial nerve
• Perform an Allen's test

EXAMINATION OF THE HANDS

1. Introduce yourself and ask permission to examine

2. Look

▸ Say what you see!
▸ ensure adequate exposure with sleeves up to elbows.
▸ ask the patient to rest his/her hands on a pillow/desk

Check the posture and the position of the hand (cascade, clawing and rotation).

Note: In normal functional position, the cascade of the hand should be one where the digits are flexed at the MCPJ and both IPJs, more so on the ulnar side rather than the radial side (**Figure 4.1**).

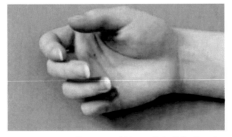

Figure 4.1: The normal 'Cascade' of the hand

Kean J, Stephen C, Hughes J, Enoch S. Focused Clinical Examination for MRCS Finals (OSCE). Doctors Academy Publications

Start with any obvious or striking abnormalities. Then ensure a systematic approach, e.g., distal to proximal / dorsal to volar.

Inspect the following and mention any positive findings.

- Scars
- Nails and nail folds
- Digits – nodules, joint deformities or subluxation
- Hand – skin quality, bruising, discolouration, rashes, muscle wasting.

Ask the patient to turn his/her hands over and look at the volar aspect.

Again start with the pulps of the fingers and work down the digits looking for any deformities or abnormal positioning of the fingers.

- Scars
- Nodules
- Contractures
- Pits/Bands/Cords
- Palmar erythema
- Muscle wasting especially in the thenar / hypothenar eminences

Also inspect the forearms and elbows for scars, nodules and skin conditions

3. Feel

Ask the patient if there is a specific area of pain or discomfort

Assess the capillary return (normal is less than 2 secs), pulses and consider Allen's test to assess for compromised circulation in the palm suggestive of a radial or ulnar artery pathology.

(For description of Allen's test – see CHAPTER 10: PERIPHERAL VASCULAR SYSTEM 2 – UPPER LIMB)

Assess skin quality

Assess temperature – use the dorsum of your hand to feel the temperature on both the dorsal and volar aspects of the patient's hand. Compare this with the other side.

Gently bimanually palpate along all joints from distal to proximal including all DIPJ, PIPJ and MCPJs paying particular attention to any joints that appear swollen, warm or tender.

Feel for bony swellings such as squaring of CMC joint of the thumb and Heberden's or Bouchard's nodes

Feel the muscle bulk in the thenar and the hypothenar eminences, and compare it with the other side

Feel for any evidence of Dupuytren's disease such as contracture, bands, cords and nodules.

4. Move

Briefly assess the patient's active movement by asking them to fully straighten all fingers and then make a fist.
Assess flexor and extensor function in each digit - if the patient is unable to undertake an active movement, try to elicit a passive movement.

Remember to test separately for both sets of flexor tendons

Flexor digitorum profundus - stabilise the PIPJ and ask the patient to flex at the DIPJ (**Figure 4.2**).

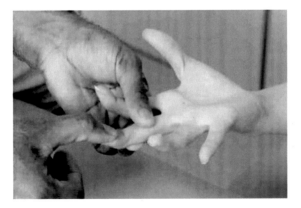

Figure 4.2: Testing for Flexor Digitorum Profundus function

Flexor digitorum superficialis, isolate the finger being examined by holding the other fingers in extension, then ask the patient to flex at the PIPJ (**Figure 4.3**).

Kean J, Stephen C, Hughes J, Enoch S. Focused Clinical Examination for MRCS Finals (OSCE). Doctors Academy Publications

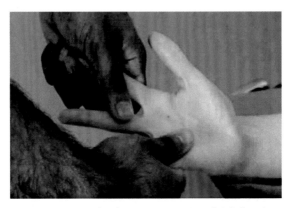

Figure 4.3: Testing for Flexor Digitorum Superficialis function

Assess all movements of the thumb – flexion, extension, abduction, adduction and opposition

NB: To simply check for extension of the thumb, ask the patient to place his/her hand palm down on the table and see if he/she are able to raise his/her thumb off the table. Feel for integrity of the Extensor Pollicis Longus tendon. *(In conditions such as Rheumatoid arthritis or post-Colles' fracture, the Extensor Pollicis Longus tendon may undergo attrition rupture as the tendon swings around the dorsal radial tubercle ([Lister's tubercle]).*

Finally assess functional capacity by asking the patient to:

• grip your two fingers to test for power grip
• pinch your finger to test for pincer grip
• pick up a small object; this will test for pincer grip and function
• pick up a pen and write
• hold a glass or a cup

5. Neurological assessment of the hand

Consider specific assessment of the functional integrity of the major nerves

Median Nerve: Supplies "LOAF" i.e., lumbricals (radial two), opponens pollicis, abductor pollicis brevis and flexor pollicis brevis

Therefore to simply test the median nerve motor function ask the patient to abduct the thumb ("lift the thumb towards the ceiling") and oppose it against the little finger (ideally without opposing the little finger concurrently).

If there is any loss of median nerve function, evaluate for any evidence of carpal tunnel syndrome including Phalens and Tinel's tests

Phalens test – passively hyperflex the patient's wrists and hold in that position for up to a minute. The test is positive if the patient's reports numbness, tingling or pain in the distribution of the median nerve (**Figure 4.4**).

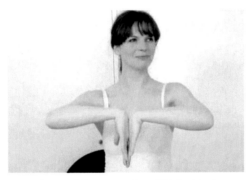

Figure 4.4: Demonstration of Phalen's test

Tinel's test – tap lightly over the carpal tunnel. Again the test is positive if the patient reports numbness, tingling or pain in the distribution of the median nerve (**Figure 4.5**).

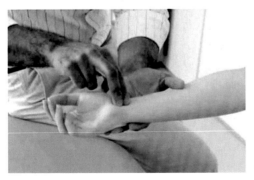

Figure 4.5: Demonstration of Tinel's test

Kean J, Stephen C, Hughes J, Enoch S. Focused Clinical Examination for MRCS Finals (OSCE). Doctors Academy Publications

Ulnar Nerve: Supplies all other intrinsic muscles of the hand

To simply test the ulnar nerve motor function, ask the patient to cross or "scissor" their index and middle fingers together. This assesses abduction and adduction. Remember "PAD and DAB"

Palmar interossei – adduct the fingers (**Figure 4.6**)

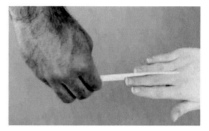

Figure 4.6: Testing for the action of Palmar interossei

Dorsal interossei – abduct the fingers (**Figure 4.7**)

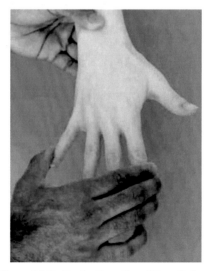

Figure 4.7: Testing for the action of Dorsal interossei

Kean J, Stephen C, Hughes J, Enoch S. Focused Clinical Examination for MRCS Finals (OSCE). Doctors Academy Publications

Also test for **Froment's sign** - ask the patient to grasp a piece of paper between the index finger and the thumb. You then try to pull the paper away. If there is an ulnar nerve lesion, the distal phalanx of the thumb flexes (due to action of the unaffected flexor pollicis longus) to compensate for the weak muscle (adductor pollicis) that is supplied by the ulnar nerve. This is a positive Froment's sign (**Figure 4.8**).

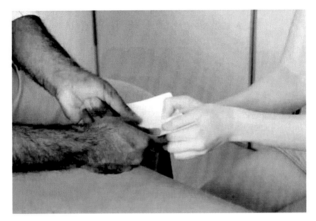

Figure 4.8: Demonstration of Froment's test, positive on the right

Radial Nerve: Supplies all the muscles in the extensor compartment.

To simply test radial nerve motor function ask the patient to extend the fingers and wrist against resistance.

Assess the patient's sensation in regions corresponding to radial, median and ulnar innervation. Note the autonomous areas for each nerve (**Figure 4.9**, **Figure 4.10** and **Figure 4.11**).

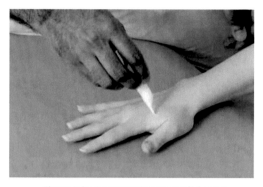

Figure 4.9: Autonomous zone: Radial nerve

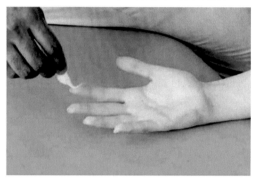

Figure 4.10: Autonomous zone: Median nerve

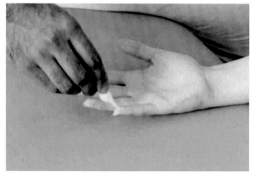

Figure 4.11: Autonomous zone: Ulnar nerve

Say you would test for light touch and pinprick, as well as 2-point discrimination.

Kean J, Stephen C, Hughes J, Enoch S. Focused Clinical Examination for
MRCS Finals (OSCE). Doctors Academy Publications

6. To complete the examination:

- Examine the rest of the upper limb as appropriate
- Look at relevant radiographs
- Consider special studies e.g. nerve conduction studies.

7. Thank the patient

IMPORTANT TIPS WHILE EXAMINING A HAND:

1. The hand pathologies could be either:

   a. Due to local causes, or

   b. Manifestation of an underlying systemic disorder

2. You need to have a clear plan/system for examination

3. Either go from distal to proximal, or from proximal to distal

4. Look at both volar and dorsal sides

5. Look and feel at both hands

6. Remember: LOOK, FEEL and MOVE

7. Think of the anatomical structures in the hand that you are examining:

   a. Nail/nail bed

   b. Skin

   c. Subcutaneous tissue

   d. Palmar fascia

   e. Tendon

   f. Joint/synovium

   g. Bone

8. The examination of the hand is never ever complete unless you have assessed

the sensory and motor functions, and the vascular status

Kean J, Stephen C, Hughes J, Enoch S. Focused Clinical Examination for
MRCS Finals (OSCE). Doctors Academy Publications

BE PREPARED TO ANSWER QUESTIONS ON:

- Duputyren's disease
- Arthritis – OA/RA and psoriotic arthropathy
- Trigger finger
- Ganglions
- Mallet finger
- Features of Rheumatoid hand
- Management of Rheumatoid hand
- Ulna nerve lesions and the concept of the ulna paradox
- Median neve lesions and carpal tunnel syndrome
- Radial nerve lesions
- Clinical anatomy of brachial plexus and lesions

Exercise Page

CHAPTER 5

HIP

POSSIBLE QUESTIONS YOU MAY GET ASKED:

• Assess this patient's hip
• Assess this patient's limb length
• Perform Trendelenburg test on this patient
• Assess this patient for a fixed flexion deformity or perform Thomas test on this patient

EXAMINATION OF THE HIP JOINT

1. Introduce yourself and ask permission to examine

2. Inspect with patient standing up

Look from front, sides and back for:

• Scars, sinuses
• Swelling, inflammation
• Gluteal wasting
• Deformity
• Pelvic tilt
• Increased lumbar lordosis, scoliosis
• Accessories, e.g., walking stick

3. Assess gait

Ask the patient whether he/she uses any walking aids. Then ask him/her to walk across the room and back.

4. Trendelenburg test (Negative if opposite hip rises, positive if falls)

Get the patient to place his/her hands on yours. Ask him/her to stand on each leg in turn. Look for pelvic movement on the opposite side. Note any pressure on your hands (Figure 5.1).

Kean J, Stephen C, Hughes J, Enoch S. Focused Clinical Examination for MRCS Finals (OSCE). Doctors Academy Publications

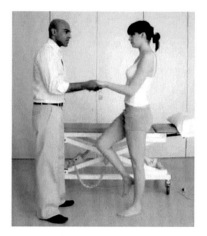

Figure 5.1 : Demonstration of the Trendelenberg test

The test is negative if the pelvis tilts upwards on the opposite side (this is normal)

The test is positive if the pelvis tilts downwards on the opposite side

5. With patient lying on couch

a) Look

• Check whether the Anterior Superior Iliac Spines (ASIS) are at the same level

• Look at the ankle alignment (any obvious difference in leg length?)

• Look at position of patella and foot on each side (for external rotation)

• Look at the angle between thigh and bed (any fixed flexion deformity?)

THOMAS TEST – Assesses fixed flexion deformity. With the examiner's hand behind patient's back, ask him/her to fully flex the opposite hip and feel for obliteration of lumbar lordosis. Whilst the lumbar lordosis is being obliterated, the patient should be able to keep the hip fully extended on the side being tested. Thomas test is positive if this hip flexes. In this case, the degree of flexion should be measured (**Figure 5.2**).

Kean J, Stephen C, Hughes J, Enoch S. Focused Clinical Examination for MRCS Finals (OSCE). Doctors Academy Publications

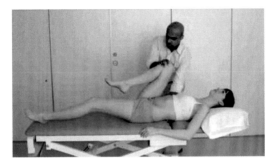

Figure 5.2: Demonstration of the Thomas test to evaluate for fixed flexion deformity

b) Feel

- ▶ Ask the patient if there is any area (s) of localised pain
- ▶ Compare the temperature using the dorsum of your hand
- ▶ Palpate over greater trochanter for tenderness
- ▶ Feel over the anterior joint line (just lateral to femoral pulse)

c) Measure

1. Apparent leg length: From xiphisternum or umbilicus to medial malleolus (**Figure 5.3**)

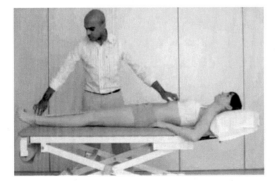

Figure 5.3: Measuring the leg length from the xiphisternum to the medial malleolus

2. True leg length: From ASIS to medial malleolus (**Figure 5.4**)

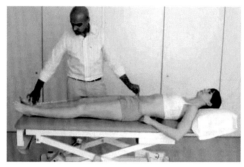

Figure 5.4: Measuring the leg length from the ASIS to the medial malleolus

If any disparity is noted, then look for femoral shortening:

Ask patient to flex knees, keeping ankles together and compare the position of the knees
If there is shortening above the knee, you can measure the distance from the ASIS to the greater trochanter (put thumbs on ASISs and feel down with fingers until you reach top of greater trochanters)
A difference in distance suggests that the shortening is in the hip joint itself.

d) Move

Test active and passive movements:
• Flexion
• Internal and external rotation with hip and knee flexed to 90º
• Abduction and adduction
  ▸ Make sure that the ASISs remain aligned
Consider assessing extension of the hip with patient prone but this is not usually required if Thomas test has already been undertaken.

6. To complete the examination

• Examine the back and knees
• Perform a neurological and vascular examination of the lower limb
• Perform an X-ray of the hip (or request relevant radiological investigation)

7. Thank the patient

Kean J, Stephen C, Hughes J, Enoch S. Focused Clinical Examination for
MRCS Finals (OSCE). Doctors Academy Publications

BE PREPARED TO ANSWER QUESTIONS ON:

- Arthritis of the hip including RA and OA – know the differences in symptoms/ examination findings and X-Ray findings
- Various options for treating OA hip – including conservative/surgical options (resurfacing vs. total hip replacement)
- Different surgical approaches to the hip joint
- Assessment, classification and management of fractured neck of femur, and complications
- Avascular necrosis and blood supply to the head of the femur
- **OA HIP:** Antalgic gait, positive Trendelenberg test, positive Thomas test. Shorter apparent limb length on affected side, affected hip lies in external rotation/ adduction. Tender over greater trochanter. Restricted range of movements, especially rotation. X-Ray: "LOSS" – Loss of joint space, Osteophytes, Subchondral cysts, Subchondral sclerosis. Possible treatment options – conservative (medical) vs. surgical (including resurfacing, hemiarthroplasty and total hip replacement.)
- **RA HIP:** Antalgic gait, gluteal and thigh wasting, held in external rotation and fixed flexion (positive Thomas test); restricted and painful range of movements.
  X-Ray: progressive bony erosion without osteophytes
- **POST-OP THR:** Scars – remember different approaches to the hip. Otherwise can be essentially normal exam. Be careful with assessing rotation as this can occasionally cause dislocation
- **Surgical approaches to the hip** – anterior, anterolateral, lateral, posterior
- **? # NOF:** You will not get a patient with an acute # NOF but may get asked to review an X-Ray -
  - ▸ Gardens classification
  - ▸ Subsequent management options – cannulated screws vs. DHS vs. hemiarthroplasty vs. THR
  - ▸ Complications

Kean J, Stephen C, Hughes J, Enoch S. Focused Clinical Examination for MRCS Finals (OSCE). Doctors Academy Publications

Exercise Page

CHAPTER 6

KNEE

1. Introduce yourself and ask permission to examine

2. Inspect with patient standing up

Look for:

• Swelling: pre-patellar / infra-patellar
• Scars
• Muscle wasting
• Erythema
• Deformities (valgus and varus)
• Asymmetry
• Baker's Cyst in Popliteal Fossa
• Accessories, e.g., walking stick / crutches

3. Observe gait

Ask the patient whether he/she uses any walking aids, then ask him/her to walk across the room and back

4. With patient lying on couch

a) Look

• Deformities (varus/valgus)
• Deviation of patella

Kean J, Stephen C, Hughes J, Enoch S. Focused Clinical Examination for
MRCS Finals (OSCE). Doctors Academy Publications

b) Feel

- Ask the patient if there are any areas of localized pain
- Temperature
  ▸ Compare both sides using dorsum of hand
- Tenderness along the joint line and popliteal fossa
  ▸ Ask patient to flex his/her knees to 90º
  ▸ Feel joint line, collateral ligaments and attachments, tibial tubercle and femoral condyles
- Test for effusions, with the knee relaxed in extension:

  ▸ *Bulge/massage/fluid displacement test* - Firmly massage fluid from the medial knee, over the superior border of the patella, on to the lateral aspect of the knee. Following this, quickly and firmly sweep your hand down the lateral knee. The test is positive if you see a fluid thrill re-filling the antero-medial aspect of the knee (**Figure 6.1**).

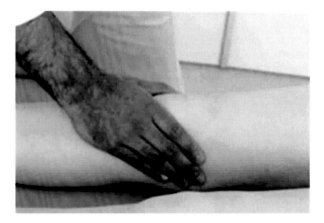

Figure 6.1: Demonstration of Bulge/massage/fluid displacement test

▶ *Patellar tap* - Standing on the patient's right, use your left hand to firmly push down from the mid-thigh to the superior border of the patella. With the patella firmly supported, tap briskly with your right hand. The test is positive if you feel obvious fluctuance or if you hear a tap as the patella bounces off the femur (**Figure 6.2**).

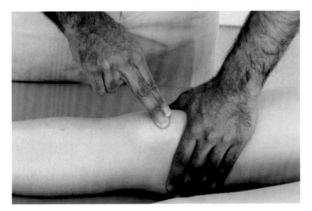

Figure 6.2: Demonstration of Patellar tap test

c) **Measure thigh circumference**

For quadriceps wasting (at fixed point above tibial tuberosity, or 10cm above upper pole of patella) (**Figure 6.3**)

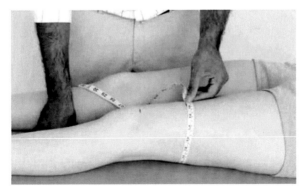

Figure 6.3: Measuring the thigh circumference for quadriceps wasting

Kean J, Stephen C, Hughes J, Enoch S. Focused Clinical Examination for MRCS Finals (OSCE). Doctors Academy Publications

d) Move

Test active movement first, if restricted then test passive movements

• Flexion (remember to feel for crepitus)
• Extension and hyperextension
• Straight leg raise

e) Special tests

• Anterior and posterior draw test

▸ With the patient's knees flexed, sit on his/her feet and move each lower leg forwards and backwards looking for excess movement and posterior sag (**Figure 6.4** and **Figure 6.5**)

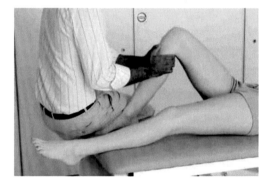

Figure 6.4: Demonstration of Anterior draw test

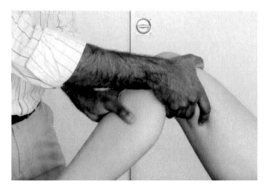

Figure 6.5: Demonstration of Posterior draw test

Kean J, Stephen C, Hughes J, Enoch S. Focused Clinical Examination for MRCS Finals (OSCE). Doctors Academy Publications

▸ This tests the stability of the anterior and posterior cruciate ligaments

▸ You can also check cruciate stability with the **Lachman test**, but only if you have large hands! Hold the thigh posteriorly and the leg anteriorly, stressing the joint by pushing inwards to check the posterior cruciate ligament. Reverse your hands, holding the thigh anteriorly and the leg posteriorly, stressing the joint by pushing inwards to check the anterior cruciate ligament.

• **Test the Collateral ligaments**

▸ With the knee flexed at 30º, put stress on the medial and lateral joint line. Look for ligamental laxity (**Figure 6.6** and **Figure 6.7**).

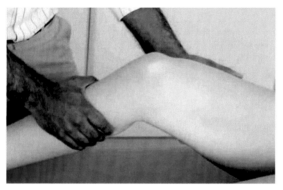

Figure 6.6: Testing the medial collateral ligament

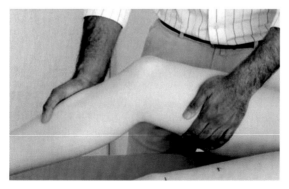

Figure 6.7: Testing the lateral collateral ligament

Kean J, Stephen C, Hughes J, Enoch S. Focused Clinical Examination for MRCS Finals (OSCE). Doctors Academy Publications

- **Offer to do McMurray's test or the pivot shift test for rotational instability**
  - ▸ These are often uncomfortable and not normally performed on patients in the exam
  - ▸ *McMurray's test* - Standing on the patient's right, hold the foot in your right hand and place your left hand over the anteromedial aspect of the knee. Lift the leg, flexing the knee and abducting and internally rotating the hip. The test is positive for meniscal injury if you feel clicks or grating under your left hand (**Figure 6.8**)

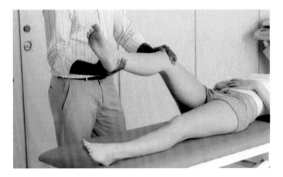

Figure 6.8: Demonstration of McMurray's test

  - ▸ *Pivot shift test* - Hold the leg internally rotated and in a valgus position, with the foot tucked under your arm. Flex then extend the knee, looking for the femoral condyle jerking forwards and backwards (**Figure 6.9**).

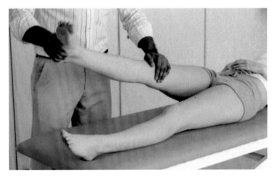

Figure 6.9: Demonstration of Pivot shift test

Kean J, Stephen C, Hughes J, Enoch S. Focused Clinical Examination for MRCS Finals (OSCE). Doctors Academy Publications

5. To complete the examination

Say you would also like to

- Examine the hip
- Perform a complete neurovascular examination of the lower limb
- Review any relevant radiology

6. Thank the patient

Kean J, Stephen C, Hughes J, Enoch S. Focused Clinical Examination for
MRCS Finals (OSCE). Doctors Academy Publications

BE PREPARED TO ANSWER QUESTIONS ON:

- Arthritis – OA causes varus deformity, RA causes valgus deformity
- Cruciate and collateral ligaments
- Signs of meniscal injury
- Causes and signs of common peroneal nerve injury
- Indications for knee replacement
- Types of knee replacement

Kean J, Stephen C, Hughes J, Enoch S. Focused Clinical Examination for
MRCS Finals (OSCE). Doctors Academy Publications

CHAPTER 7

NECK

POSSIBLE QUESTIONS YOU MAY GET ASKED:

• Examine this patient's neck

• Examine this neck lump

• Examine this patient's lymph nodes

EXAMINATION OF THE NECK

1. Introduce yourself and ask permission to examine

2. Adequately expose the neck – Move the patient if required

3. Inspect - From front and side

Look for

• General condition of patient - cachectic?
• Obvious neck lumps / swellings or asymmetry
• Scars
• Post radiotherapy skin changes e.g., telangectasia
• Facial asymmetry, e.g., post-surgical palsy

NB: Observe around the bay for a cup of water which may indicate this is a thyroid examination.

If unsure, start by asking for a cup of water and asking the patient to swallow/ protrude their tongue. If this is not a thyroid examination the examiners will move you along otherwise proceed with the thyroid examination as described in CHAPTER 13: THYROID.

4. Move behind the patient and systematically palpate the neck

• Remember to warn the patient that you are about to start palpating his/her neck and ask for any pain or tenderness.

• Feel for presence of any lumps / lymph nodes in the neck ensuring you systematically cover both the anterior and posterior triangles.

Kean J, Stephen C, Hughes J, Enoch S. Focused Clinical Examination for MRCS Finals (OSCE). Doctors Academy Publications

Remember to specifically palpate the following regions:

- Submental
- Submandibular
- Parotid / Pre-auricular
- Post-auricular
- Occipital
- Superficial and deep cervical chains
- Supraclavicular
- Midline for thyroid

For any palpable neck lumps comment on:

- Size
- Mobility in relation to underlying structures
- Consistency (hard/firm/rubbery), nodularity, fluctuance
- Tenderness

5. To complete the examination:

Say you would also like to assess the:

- Tracheal position
- Oral cavity and aerodigestive tract ± flexible nasal endoscopy
- Voice and vocal cord function
- Cutaneous lesions on the face / scalp

6. Thank the patient

BE PREPARED TO ANSWER QUESTIONS ON:

- Causes of cervical lymphadenopathy
- Other causes of neck swellings, e.g., branchial cysts, carotid body tumours, cystic hygromas, pharyngeal pouch
- How would you investigate a neck lump?
- What are the causes of airway obstruction?
- How would you secure an airway in an emergency?
- How would you perform a cricothyroidectomy?
- Tracheostomies – know the basic technique for the procedure.

Kean J, Stephen C, Hughes J, Enoch S. Focused Clinical Examination for MRCS Finals (OSCE). Doctors Academy Publications

Exercise Page

CHAPTER 7

PAROTID

EXAMINATION OF THE PAROTID

1. Introduce yourself and ask permission to examine

2. Inspect – from front and side

Look for

• How is the general appearance of the patient and the nutritional status?
• Are there any obvious lumps / swellings or asymmetry?
• Scars or fistulae
• Post radiotherapy skin changes, e.g., telangiectasia
• Any signs or evidence of facial asymmetry

3. Palpate

• Remember to warn the patient that you are about to start palpating his/her cheek (parotid gland) and ask for any pain or tenderness.
• Move behind the patient and feel for presence of any lumps around the cheek/angle of the jaw

Describe any lump in terms of:

• Site - unilateral or bilateral
• Size

- Shape
- Edges / Surface
- Consistency / Nodularity
- Fluctuance
- Compressibility
- Reducibility
- Fixity / Tethering

Note any overlying or surrounding skin changes and any tenderness of the lump.

4. Intraoral examination

Look inside the mouth and sweep a gloved finger along the inside the cheek to feel for any stones in the parotid duct.

NB: The parotid duct opens into a papilla the level of the second upper molar. Palpate the parotid gland bimanually to fully assess for lumps or swelling (**Figure 8.1**)

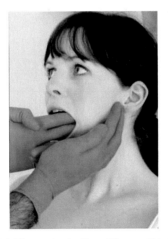

Figure 8.1: Bimanual palpation of the parotid gland

Kean J, Stephen C, Hughes J, Enoch S. Focused Clinical Examination for MRCS Finals (OSCE). Doctors Academy Publications

5. Assess facial nerve function

Test muscles systematically

- Temporal branch (occipitofrontalis) – "raise your eyebrows" (**Figure 8.2**)

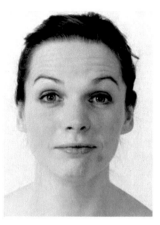

Figure 8.2: Examining the *temporal branch* of the facial nerve: ***"Raise your eyebrows"***

- Zygomatic branch (orbicularis oris) – "close your eyes tightly" (**Figure 8.3**)

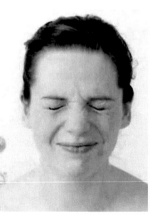

Figure 8.3: Examining the *zygomatic branch* of the facial nerve: *"**Close your eyes tightly"***

Kean J, Stephen C, Hughes J, Enoch S. Focused Clinical Examination for
MRCS Finals (OSCE). Doctors Academy Publications

- Buccal branch (buccinator) – "puff out your cheeks" (**Figure 8.4**)

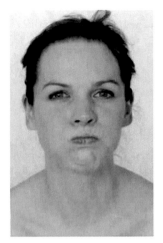

Figure 8.4: Examining the *buccal branch* of the facial nerve: ***"Puff out your cheeks"***

- Marginal mandibular branch (orbicularis oris) – "show me your teeth" (**Figure 8.5**)

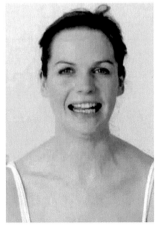

Figure 8.5: Examining the *marginal mandibular branch* of the facial nerve: ***"Show me your teeth"***

Kean J, Stephen C, Hughes J, Enoch S. Focused Clinical Examination for MRCS Finals (OSCE). Doctors Academy Publications

• Cervical branch – "tense your neck muscles" (**Figure 8.6**)

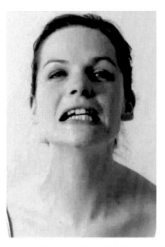

Figure 8.6: Examining the *cervical branch* of the facial nerve: ***"Tense your neck muscles"***

6. To complete the examination

• Feel for other salivary gland swellings
• Examine the regional lymph nodes as for any neck lump
• Perform a full ENT examination

7. Thank the patient

Kean J, Stephen C, Hughes J, Enoch S. Focused Clinical Examination for
MRCS Finals (OSCE). Doctors Academy Publications

BE PREPARED TO ANSWER QUESTIONS ON:

• Anatomy of the parotid gland and course of the facial nerve passing through it

• Intra-cranial and extra-cranial course of the facial nerve and its branches

• Causes of parotid lumps

• Management of a parotid lump

• Basic principles of parotidectomy and complications

• Facial nerve palsy

• Salivary stones (sialolithiasis)

Kean J, Stephen C, Hughes J, Enoch S. Focused Clinical Examination for
MRCS Finals (OSCE). Doctors Academy Publications

CHAPTER 9

PERIPHERAL VASCULAR SYSTEM 1

EXAMINATION OF THE PERIPHERAL VASCULAR SYSTEM

1. Introduce yourself and ask permission to examine

2. Inspect (with the patient lying on the couch):

general:

- Observe the patient and the surroundings from the end of the bed
- Look for any evidence of obvious signs of cardiovascular disease, e.g., bypass scars, GTN spray
- Inspect the hands looking for nicotine staining, tendon xanthomata, nail fold infarcts and splinter haemorrhages and nail changes
- Look at the skin and hair for changes suggestive of arterial disease, i.e., thin/shiny skin and hair loss.

Specific:

Look at the legs for

- Colour of the legs -do they appear pale, cyanosed or red?
- Scars suggestive of previous surgery (e.g., femoro-distal bypass) or amputated digits
- Signs of venous insufficiency such as lipodermatosclerosis, venous eczema and atrophy blanche

Kean J, Stephen C, Hughes J, Enoch S. Focused Clinical Examination for MRCS Finals (OSCE). Doctors Academy Publications

- Venous guttering - seen when veins collapse in limbs with peripheral vascular disease and appear as shallow grooves
- Ulceration - comment on the location, shape depth and size of the ulcer

NB: Arterial ulcers typically have a "punched out" appearance and are generally found around pressure areas, i.e., lateral and medial malleoli, tips of the toes, head of the 1st and 5th metatarsals, the heel and the interdigital clefts – so remember to look between toes and under the heel.

(May often be confused with neuropathic ulceration; venous ulceration commonly occurs around the gaiter region (medial side) of the leg)

- Gangrene

3. Palpation:

- Compare the temperature on both legs using the dorsum of your hand.

- Check the capillary refill time in toes of both feet. (*NB:* normal = <2 sec)

- Say you would like to perform **BUERGERS TEST**

  ▸ With the patient lying supine, ask if they have any pain or restriction in hip movements. Then lift both legs slowly (ideally in about 10 degree increments and waiting for 10 seconds at each stage) and evaluate the angle at which the leg becomes pale or white (**Figure 9.1**). This is known as *Buerger's angle* – in normal subjects it should be greater than 90 degrees (even if the limb is flexed further at the hip, there should be no colour change in the limb). In patients with peripheral vascular disease, the limb may go pale as it is lifted and reaches a certain angle. If the angle is less than 25-30 degrees, it suggests severe ischemia.

  ▸ You will usually also see evidence of venous guttering as you are performing this test which you should comment on.

Kean J, Stephen C, Hughes J, Enoch S. Focused Clinical Examination for MRCS Finals (OSCE). Doctors Academy Publications

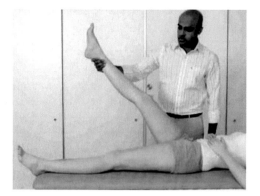

Figure 9.1: Buerger's test: Elevation of the leg in increments (about 10 degrees each time and wait for 10 seconds) and watch for pallor

▶ Once you have established Buerger's angle, sit the patient up and swing the legs over the side of the couch. Watch for the foot to reperfuse (**Figure 9.2**) – in normal subjects there should be no colour change but in patients with peripheral vascular disease, you will observe the legs becoming a dusky crimson/purple colour, which is caused by reactive hyperaemia. This represents a positive Buerger's test.

Note the time taken to achieve venous filling and establish reactive hyperaemia.

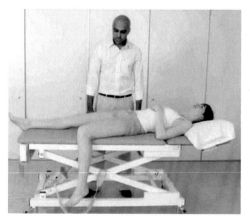

Figure 9.2: Buerger's test: Watching for dependent reperfusion and reactive hyperaemia

Kean J, Stephen C, Hughes J, Enoch S. Focused Clinical Examination for MRCS Finals (OSCE). Doctors Academy Publications

Palpate the pulses on both legs:

▸ **Femoral** – felt in the *mid-inguinal point*, halfway between the pubic symphysis and ASIS.

▸ **Popliteal** – felt deep in the midline of the popliteal fossa with the knee flexed to ~30 degrees (**Figure 9.3**).

NB: The popliteal artery is the deepest structure in the popliteal fossa therefore can be difficult to feel.

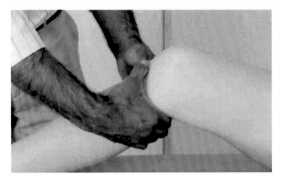

Figure 9.3: Peripheral pulses: Palpation of the popliteal artery

▸ **Posterior tibial** – felt posterior to medial malleolus, 2/3rd of the way between the medial malleolus and the insertion of the Achilles tendon (**Figure 9.4**).

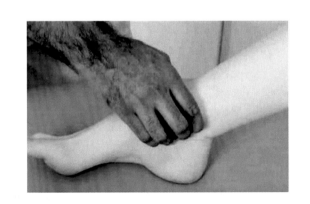

Figure 9.4: Peripheral pulses: Palpation of the posterior tibial artery

Kean J, Stephen C, Hughes J, Enoch S. Focused Clinical Examination for MRCS Finals (OSCE). Doctors Academy Publications

▶ **Dorsalis pedis** - felt in the 1st webspace, just lateral to the extensor hallucis longus tendon on the dorsal surface of the foot (dorsiflexion of the hallux may aid palpation) (**Figure 9.5**).

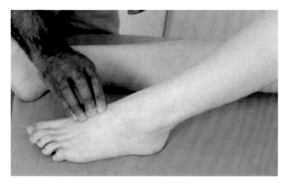

Figure 9.5: Peripheral pulses: Palpation of the dorsalis pedis artery

If unable to palpate pulses clinically say you would like to use a Doppler Ultrasound (**Figure 9.6**).

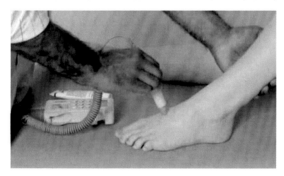

Figure 9.6 : Use of Doppler probe to assess dorsalis pedis pulsation

NB: The normal arterial signal is *triphasic*

▶ 1st phase characterised by the initial forward rush of blood from the heart
▶ 2nd phase characterised by the reverse flow caused by the elastic recoil of the artery wall
▶ 3rd phase characterised by the forward flow once the vessel has relaxed.

In arterial disease there is a loss of reverse flow so the signal becomes *biphasic*. If there is severe stenosis, the signal may become even more damped, thus only a *monophasic* signal is heard.

Remember also to check the radial pulse and assess for radio-femoral delay.

NB: The normal arterial signal is *triphasic*

‣ 1st phase characterised by the initial forward rush of blood from the heart
‣ 2nd phase characterised by the reverse flow caused by the elastic recoil of the artery wall
‣ 3rd phase characterised by the forward flow once the vessel has relaxed.

In arterial disease there is a loss of reverse flow so the signal becomes *biphasic*. If there is severe stenosis, the signal may become even more damped, thus only a *monophasic* signal is heard.

Remember also to check the radial pulse and assess for radio-femoral delay.

$$ABPI = \frac{\text{Ankle Systolic Pressure}}{\text{Brachial Systolic Pressure}}$$

The ABPI gives an indication of the severity of peripheral vascular disease where present. A normal ABPI is >1.0

If the ABPI is:

• 0.7 – 1 = mild disease (i.e., patient may present with intermittent claudication)
• 0.5 – 0.7 = moderate disease (i.e., likely to have rest pain)
• < 0.5 – 0.3 (or absolute pressure <50mmHg) = severe disease (i.e., critical ischemia)

5. Complete the exam

Say you would like to:

• Perform a complete neurological examination of the lower limbs
• Perform a full cardiovascular examination
• Perform a vascular examination of the upper limbs
• Feel the abdomen for any evidence of an aortic aneurysm and auscultate for renal and aortic bruits.

6. Thank the patient

Kean J, Stephen C, Hughes J, Enoch S. Focused Clinical Examination for MRCS Finals (OSCE). Doctors Academy Publications

BE PREPARED TO ANSWER QUESTIONS ON:

- Discussion related to what advice you would give the patient for different ABPI readings
- Appropriate investigations for peripheral vascular disease
- Management of peripheral vascular disease including conservative, endovascular and surgical
- Indications for amputation
- Types of amputation and selection of amputation level
- Surgical principles of below knee and above knee amputations
- Prosthetic limbs

Kean J, Stephen C, Hughes J, Enoch S. Focused Clinical Examination for
MRCS Finals (OSCE). Doctors Academy Publications

Exercise Page

Kean J, Stephen C, Hughes J, Enoch S. Focused Clinical Examination for
MRCS Finals (OSCE). Doctors Academy Publications

CHAPTER 10

PERIPHERAL VASCULAR SYSTEM 2

POSSIBLE QUESTIONS YOU MAY GET ASKED:

• Examine this patient's arm / upper limb

• Look at this patient's hands

EXAMINATION OF THE PERIPHERAL VASCULAR SYSTEM

1. Introduce yourself and ask permission to examine.

Ensure adequate exposure of both upper limbs – you may need to ask the patient to remove his/her top.

2. Inspect

GENERAL:

Observe the patient and his/her surroundings from the end of the bed.
Look for any evidence of obvious signs of cardiovascular disease e.g. bypass scars, GTN spray.
Look at the skin and hair for changes suggestive of arterial disease i.e. thin/shiny skin and hair loss.

SPECIFIC:

Inspect the hands for:
- Colour – pallor, cyanosis or erythema
- Skin changes including nicotine staining
- Nail changes including nail fold infarcts and splinter haemorrhages.
- Clubbing or tendon xanthomata
- Vasculitic lesions /necrotic areas of skin or previously amputated digits
- Wasting of the pulp of the fingers or small muscles of the hand

Kean J, Stephen C, Hughes J, Enoch S. Focused Clinical Examination for MRCS Finals (OSCE). Doctors Academy Publications

Inspect the arms for:
- Signs of oedema
- Scars suggestive of previous surgery (e.g., axillo-femoral bypass)

3. Palpation:

Compare the temperature of both hands using the dorsum of your hand.
Check the capillary refill time in fingers of both hands. (*NB:* normal = <2 sec)
Feel for the radial pulse bilaterally and compare for radial-radial delay
Feel for the radial pulses bilaterally whilst applying gentle traction on the shoulder

Say you would like to perform **ALLEN'S TEST:**

Identify the ulnar and radial pulsations. Ask the patient to elevate the hand and make a fist then occlude both vessels with direct pressure (**Figure 10.1**). Ask the patient to open and close his/her palm until it appears pale (**Figure 10.2**). Release the radial side and observe for reperfusion of the hand, which signifies an intact radial artery (**Figure 10.3**). Repeat for the ulnar side (**Figure 10.4**). Remember that the ulnar artery is the dominant vessel to the hand in the majority of patients.

Palpate the brachial pulse, and axillary/subclavian/carotid pulses bilaterally

Palpate around the neck, above the clavicle in the supraclavicular fossa, for evidence of a cervical rib.

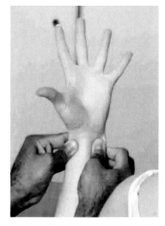

Figure 10.1: Demonstration of Allen's test: Occluding the radial and ulnar arteries

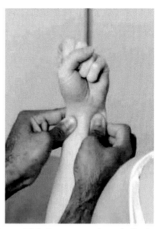

Figure 10.2: Demonstration of Allen's test: Maintaining occlusion as patient repeatedly clenches the fist

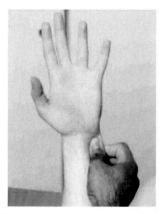

Figure 10.3: Demonstration of Allen's test: Release the radial artery and watch for reperfusion

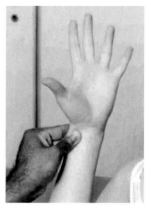

Figure 10.4: Demonstration of Allen's test: Repeat the first two steps then release the ulnar artery and watch for reperfusion

Kean J, Stephen C, Hughes J, Enoch S. Focused Clinical Examination for MRCS Finals (OSCE). Doctors Academy Publications

4. Auscultation

Listen for bruits over the carotid and subclavian arteries.

5. To complete the examination

Say you would like to:

- Measure the blood pressures in both arms
- Look at a chest X-Ray to look for a cervical rib
- Perform a complete neurological assessment of the upper limbs
- Perform a full cardiovascular examination
- Feel the abdomen for any evidence of an aortic aneurysm and auscultate for renal and aortic bruits
- Perform a full vascular assessment of the lower limbs

6. Thank the patient

Kean J, Stephen C, Hughes J, Enoch S. Focused Clinical Examination for
MRCS Finals (OSCE). Doctors Academy Publications

BE PREPARED TO ANSWER QUESTIONS ON:

Raynaud's disease

- Cervical rib / thoracic outlet obstruction
- Subclavian steal syndrome
- Axillary vein thrombosis
- Anatomical landmarks for obtaining central venous access through the axillary

  vein

Kean J, Stephen C, Hughes J, Enoch S. Focused Clinical Examination for
MRCS Finals (OSCE). Doctors Academy Publications

Exercise Page

Kean J, Stephen C, Hughes J, Enoch S. Focused Clinical Examination for
MRCS Finals (OSCE). Doctors Academy Publications

CHAPTER 11

SHOULDER

POSSIBLE QUESTIONS YOU MAY GET ASKED:

• Examine this patient's shoulder
• Examine for painful arc syndrome
• Examine for signs of rotator cuff injury

1. Introduce yourself and ask permission to examine

2. Inspect with patient standing

Look from the front, sides and behind for

• Scars
• Sinuses
• Erythema
• Joint or bony prominences
• Muscle asymmetry or deltoid wasting
• Abnormal posture

3. Feel

Ask about pain first
• Palpate the sternoclavicular joint, clavicle, coracoid process, the acromioclavicular joint, and around the glenohumeral joint.
• Palpate the spine of the scapula, the scapula borders and the surrounding muscles.
• Palpate the head of the humerus via the axilla.

4. Move

It is normally best to demonstrate the movements to the patient when assessing active movements

- Flexion and extension- ask the patient to move his/her arms up from the side with thumbs pointing upwards in front of them to above the head and then down behind the back
- Abduction and adduction- ask the patient to raise his/her hands above his/her head out to the sides in abduction and then ask them to move his/her arm directly across chest to assess adduction.
- Internal and external rotation- ask the patient to put their arms behind his/her back with his/her thumbs upwards to assess internal rotation and then ask him/her to put his/her arms behind the head and push his/her elbows backwards to assess external rotation.

Normal range of movements:

- Flexion- 180 degrees
- Extension- 50 degrees
- Abduction- 180 degrees
- Adduction- 45 degrees
- External rotation- 90 degrees
- Internal rotation- 90 degrees

5. Special tests

Examine the rotator cuff muscles:

- Supraspinatus - resisted abduction from zero degrees (**Figure 11.1**)
- Infraspinatus - resisted external rotation (**Figure 11.2**). The patient should have his/her elbows flexed at 90 degrees close to his/her sides, one of the examiner's hands should support the elbow, the other resist the pushing out of the forearm.

Kean J, Stephen C, Hughes J, Enoch S. Focused Clinical Examination for MRCS Finals (OSCE). Doctors Academy Publications

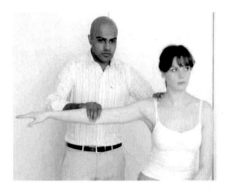

Figure 11.1: Testing for Supraspinatus: Resisted abduction from zero degrees

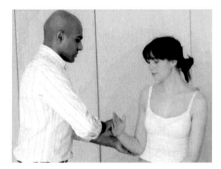

Figure 11.2: Testing for Infraspinatus: Resisted external rotation

• Subscapularis - resisted internal rotation (**Figure 11.3**). The alternative to this movement is the ***Goebers lift off test***.

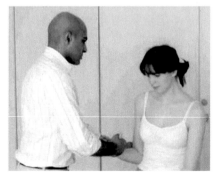

Figure 11.3: Testing for Subscapularis: Resisted internal rotation

Kean J, Stephen C, Hughes J, Enoch S. Focused Clinical Examination for MRCS Finals (OSCE). Doctors Academy Publications

Examine for winging of the scapula:

• Ask the patient to push against a wall with his/her hands outstretched at chest level (**Figure 11.4**). If the scapula is elevated like a wing this suggests damage to the long thoracic nerve.

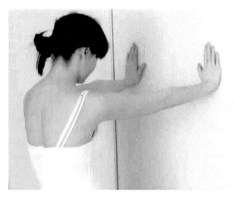

Figure 11.4: Examining for Winging of the Scapula

Examine for the lieutenant's badge sign:

• Test for light touch sensation over the lateral deltoid (**Figure 11.5**). If paraesthesia is present, this is It may indicate axillary nerve injury as occurs in anterior shoulder dislocation.

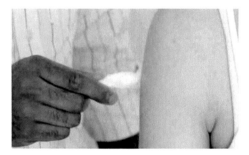

Figure 11.5: Examining for the 'Lieutenant's Badge' sign

Kean J, Stephen C, Hughes J, Enoch S. Focused Clinical Examination for MRCS Finals (OSCE). Doctors Academy Publications

Examine for the long head of biceps:

- Resisted supination of the forearm with the shoulder neutral and the elbow at 90 degrees flexion tests the long head of the biceps tendon (**Figure 11.6**).

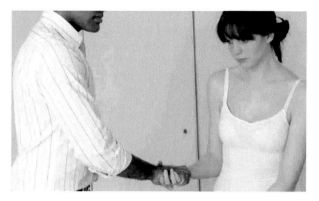

Figure 11.6: Examining for the integrity of the long head of biceps

6. To complete the examination

Say you would also like to:

- Perform a complete neurological examination of the upper limb
- Examine the neck

7. Thank the patient

Kean J, Stephen C, Hughes J, Enoch S. Focused Clinical Examination for MRCS Finals (OSCE). Doctors Academy Publications

BE PREPARED TO ANSWER QUESTIONS ON:

- Painful arc syndrome - Commonly supraspinatus tendonitis
- Frozen shoulder
- Dislocation of the shoulder - Anterior more common than posterior, may result in axillary nerve injury
- Rotator cuff injuries
- Arthritis
- Gout

Kean J, Stephen C, Hughes J, Enoch S. Focused Clinical Examination for MRCS Finals (OSCE). Doctors Academy Publications

CHAPTER 12

SUPERFICIAL LESIONS

POSSIBLE QUESTIONS YOU MAY GET ASKED:

- Assess this lesion/lump
- What is this?
- Perform a test for fluctuance

EXAMINATION OF A SUPERFICIAL LESION

1. Introduce yourself and ask permission to examine

2. Inspect with patient in good light

Look without touching, comment on

- Site
- Size (Approximate dimensions in centimetres or millimetres)
- Shape (Circular, hemispherical, flat, nodular, pedunculated, ulcerated)
- Skin surface (Pigmentation, erythema, telangiectasia, punctum, keratosis)
- Scars (Recurrent lesion?)

3. Palpate

Ask about pain first

- Assess the temperature using the dorsum of the hand
- Palpate gently and assess tenderness (look at facial expression, ask if tender)
- Feel the edges of the lesion, look for the "slip sign" – smooth edges slip away from the fingers in lipoma
- Feel the consistency of the lump (Soft, firm, hard, craggy)
- Test for fluctuance – palpate in two planes; top to bottom and left to right, parallel and perpendicular to the axis of the underlying skeletal muscle (**Figure 12.1**)

Kean J, Stephen C, Hughes J, Enoch S. Focused Clinical Examination for MRCS Finals (OSCE). Doctors Academy Publications

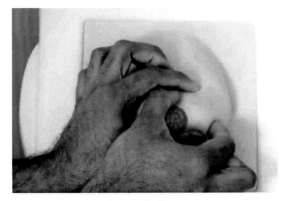

Figure 12. : Test for fluctuance

- Assess the layer from which the lesion is arising – continuous with skin, tethered to muscle, arising from muscle with skin moving freely over the lesion (ask patient to tense muscle in question, does lump become more prominent or less mobile?)
- Examine for regional lymphadenopathy (examiner may stop you due to time constraints)

4. To complete the examination

Say you would also like to:

- Take a history of the lesion - onset, duration, recent changes, other lesions, history of sun exposure, family history of skin lesions and effect on quality of life

5. Thank the patient

BE PREPARED TO ANSWER QUESTIONS ON:

- **Lipoma** – Hemispherical, normal overlying skin, non-tender, lobulated edges, slip sign, fluctuant if large, firm if small.

- **BCC** – Nodular and/or ulcerated, rolled pearly edge, telangiectasia, arising from skin, tethered if deep. This is the most common skin cancer in the UK. Locally invasive (destructive); usually doesn't metastasise.

- **SCC** – Scaly and/or ulcerated, may arise within chronic wounds (Marjolin's ulcer); may metastasise; examine for regional lymph nodes. Know the treatment options and surgical excision margins.

- **Melanoma** – Warning signs for pigmented lesion are **A**symmetry, **B**order irregular, **C**olour change, **D**iameter enlarging, **E**levation, **F**urther symptoms (itching, crusting, bleeding).

  ‣ Know the difference between Clark's level and Breslow depth

  ‣ What is the significance of Breslow depth?

  ‣ Be familiar with the different treatment options and surgical excision margins

  ‣ May be asked about sentinel node biopsy

Kean J, Stephen C, Hughes J, Enoch S. Focused Clinical Examination for MRCS Finals (OSCE). Doctors Academy Publications

Exercise Page

CHAPTER 13

THYROID

POSSIBLE QUESTIONS YOU MAY GET ASKED:

• Examine this patient's thyroid gland
• Assess this patient's thyroid status
• Examine this patient's neck

EXAMINATION OF THE THYROID

1. Introduce yourself and ask permission to examine

2. Adequately expose the neck – move the patient if required

3. Inspect - from front and side

Look for

• General condition of patient – over or underweight, appropriately dressed for current weather, agitation or listlessness?
• Any immediately obvious systemic features of thyroid disease?
• Obvious neck lumps/goitre?
• Neck scars?

4. Ask patient to swallow water

Is there a neck lump which moves upwards on swallowing?
If yes, it is likely to be of thyroid origin

5. Ask patient to protrude tongues

Is there a neck lump which moves upwards on protrusion of the tongue?
If yes, it is likely to be a thyroglossal duct cyst

6. Move behind the patient and commence palpation

Remember to warn the patient you are about to start palpation and ask about pain and tenderness.

Kean J, Stephen C, Hughes J, Enoch S. Focused Clinical Examination for MRCS Finals (OSCE). Doctors Academy Publications

a) Repeat steps 4 and 5 whilst palpating over the thyroid.

b) Feel systematically over thyroid isthmus and both lobes for presence of lumps and comment on:

- Enlargement
- Symmetry - solitary or multiple lumps
- Consistency - diffuse or nodular
- Tenderness

c) Feel for enlarged lymph nodes in the neck

d) Palpate for tracheal deviation

7. Percuss over sternum for retrosternal extension of goitre

8. Auscultate over the thyroid bilaterally for any bruits

9. To complete the examination

Say you would also like to feel for a lingual thyroid and examine for systemic features of thyroid disease.

a) Hands

- Temperature / sweating
- Clubbing / thyroid acropachy / onycholysis
- Palmar erythema
- Tremor (ask patient to stretch out hands and close eyes)

b) Radial pulse

- AF or tachycardia

c) Face

- Dry skin
- Loss or coarsening of hair
- Loss of lateral third of eyebrows
- Oedema

d) Eyes

• Lid lag and lid retraction are non-specific signs of hyperthyroidism

Ask the patient to follow your finger downwards with his/her eyes

• Ophthalmoplegia, proptosis and chemosis are pathognomonic of Grave's disease

e) Muscle power: test for proximal myopathy

• Test shoulder abduction

• Ask patient to stand up from chair without using his/her arms

f) Check reflexes (especially supinator and ankle jerks)

g) Look at the shins for pretibial myxoedema

Say you would like to arrange thyroid function tests to assess thyroid status.

10. Thank the patient

Kean J, Stephen C, Hughes J, Enoch S. Focused Clinical Examination for MRCS Finals (OSCE). Doctors Academy Publications

BE PREPARED TO ANSWER QUESTIONS ON:

- Causes of thyroid swelling – solitary nodules, multinodular goitres, diffuse thyroid enlargement
- Thyroid malignancy
- Thyrotoxicosis and Graves disease
- Hypothyroidism and myxoedema
- Treatment of thyroid disease – indications for surgery
- Complications of thyroid surgery
- Thyroglossal cysts

CHAPTER 14

VARICOSE VEINS

POSSIBLE QUESTIONS YOU MAY GET ASKED:

- Assess this patient's legs
- Examine this patient's varicose veins
- Perform Trendelenburg's test on this patient
- Perform a Tourniquet test on this patient
- Perform Perthe's test on this patient
- Demonstrate how you might assess for venous reflux using a Doppler probe

EXAMINATION OF VARICOSE VEINS:

1. Introduce yourself and ask permission to examine

2. Inspect with the patient standing up

Ensure that the patient is adequately exposed whilst dignity maintained.

Inspect from all sides - easiest done by kneeling in front of the patient then asking the patient to turn around.

Look for:

- Varicosities i.e. dilated, tortuous veins along the long and short saphenous systems

NB: Remember surface landmarks for the long saphenous and short saphenous veins as you may be expected to describe the course and this will also help establish the origin of any varicosities identified.

Long (Great) saphenous vein: Commences from the medial venous arch, runs 2 cm in front of the medial malleolus, ascends along the medial border of the tibia, runs a hand's breadth medial to the medial border of the patella, goes up the medial

Kean J, Stephen C, Hughes J, Enoch S. Focused Clinical Examination for MRCS Finals (OSCE). Doctors Academy Publications

side of the thigh, pierces the cribriform fascia and empties into the femoral vein at the sapheno-femoral junction that lies ~4 cm below and lateral (obliquely) to the pubic tubercle. The saphenous nerve, which is a continuation of the femoral nerve, accompanies the vein from the knee all the way down to the medial aspect of the foot. (Saphenous nerve provides sensation to the medial aspect of the foot).

Short saphenous vein: Commences from the lateral venous arch, runs behind the lateral malleolus, ascends along the leg lying in the midline and empties into the sapheno-popliteal junction that lies about 4-5 cm above the posterior joint line of the knee. The sural nerve accompanies the vein from the posterior aspect of the knee all the way down to the lateral aspect of the foot. (Sural nerve provides sensation to the lateral aspect of the foot).

- Skin changes and ulceration from chronic varicosities and their complications especially the medial "gaiter" area
  - Lipodermatosclerosis
  - Venous eczema
  - Haemosiderin staining
  - "Atrophie blanche" – white patches found in areas of healed ulceration
  - Oedema
- Scars from previous surgery, including avulsion scars
- Look for any evidence of sapheno varix in the groin

For extra brownie points!

Look for evidence of port-wine stains and soft tissue limb hypertrophy together with varicosities, particularly around the lateral thigh, which may be associated with congenital disorders or underlying arterio-venous malformations e.g. Klippel-Trenaunay syndrome

3. Palpation (with the patient still standing):

- Feel at the sapheno-femoral junction (~4cm below and lateral to the pubic tubercle) for a sapheno varix. If a swelling is present check for a palpable thrill and a cough impulse which indicates an incompetent valve between the superficial and deep systems

- Feel down the leg over the course of the long saphenous and then short saphenous veins for tenderness along the veins which may indicate perforator incompetence.

NB: The perforators in the long saphenous vein that are clinically important are 5, 10 and 15 cms above the medial malleolus, one a few cms below the knee joint, one a few cms above the knee joint, one in the adductor canal and one in the upper thigh.

In order to elucidate if the varicosity is due to sapheno-femoral junctional incompetence or due to perforator incompetence you may be asked to perform either the Trendelenberg test or Tourniquet test although these have been largely superseded in clinical practice by Doppler.

4. With the patient lying down

Look for the varicosities collapsing as the patient lies down. If they remain engorged, you should consider an arterio-venous fistula of physical obstruction to venous drainage rather than varicose veins.

TRENDELENBERG TEST

With the patient lying supine, lift his/her leg to about 45 degrees and gently empty the veins (this may be aided by "milking" the veins) (**Figure 14.1**).

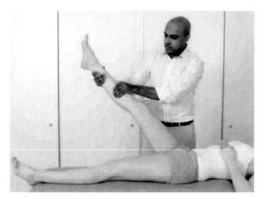

Figure 14.1: Trendelenberg test: Elevation of the to 45 degrees and milking of the veins to empty them

Kean J, Stephen C, Hughes J, Enoch S. Focused Clinical Examination for MRCS Finals (OSCE). Doctors Academy Publications

NB: It is a good idea to ask the patient for any pain or restriction in movements in the hip joint before lifting the leg.

Occlude the sapheno-femoral junction (**Figure 14.2**) and ask the patient to stand up ensuring that the finger or thumb is firmly over the junction (**Figure 14.3**).

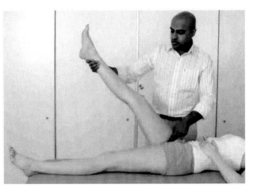

Figure 14.2: Trendelenberg test: Occlusion at the sapheno-femoral junction

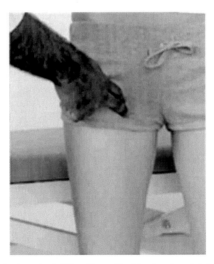

Figure 14.3: Trendelenberg test: Allow the patient to stand, maintaining occlusion of the sapheno-femoral junction, and watch for veins filling from below

Kean J, Stephen C, Hughes J, Enoch S. Focused Clinical Examination for MRCS Finals (OSCE). Doctors Academy Publications

- If the superficial veins do not fill and the varicosities are controlled at the level of the sapheno-femoral junction by occluding it, it strongly suggests sapheno-femoral incompetence. This can be confirmed by releasing the pressure from the sapheno-femoral junction that will cause the blood to return from the femoral vein into the saphenous vein (through the incompetent sapheno-femoral junction), resulting in the varicosities becoming prominent.

- As the patient stands, if the veins fill from below with the sapheno-femoral junction occluded, incompetent perforators are the most likely cause for the varicosities.

TOURNIQUET TEST

The tourniquet test follows the same principle but is easier to perform than Trendelenberg's test as it uses a tourniquet to control the sapheno-femoral junction rather than the examiner's fingers.

It also has the added advantage that if varicosities are due to perforator incompetence, it can be performed further down the leg to identify the level of the incompetence (**Figure 14.4** and **Figure 14.5**).

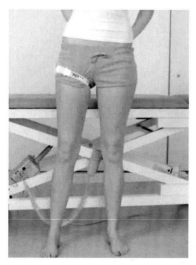

Figure 14.4: Tourniquet test: Identify the site of incompetent perforators

Kean J, Stephen C, Hughes J, Enoch S. Focused Clinical Examination for MRCS Finals (OSCE). Doctors Academy Publications

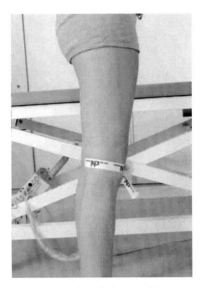

Figure 14.5: Tourniquet test: Identify the site of incompetent perforators

Once the superficial venous system has been controlled with the tourniquet you can perform Perthe's test to assess the patency of the deep venous system, particularly important if considering varicose vein surgery

PERTHE'S TEST

With the patient standing and with the tourniquet still around the thigh ask the patient to go up and down on his/her tiptoes or ask him/her to walk, thus exercising the calf muscles. If the deep venous system is intact, the calf pumps encourage venous return. However, if the deep venous system is occluded or valves incompetent, when the patient performs this action venous return is restricted and blood is forced into the superficial system from the deep system, causing engorgement of the superficial veins associated with a bursting pain.

DOPPLER ULTRASOUND

To assess for sapheno-femoral incompetence using a hand-held Doppler - hold the Doppler probe at a 45 degree angle to the skin at the level of the sapheno-femoral junction and the squeeze the patient's calf. In a patient with a competent sapheno-femoral junction you will hear a short "swoosh" as you squeeze, but this ceases as soon as you let go of the calf. If however, the sapheno-femoral junction is incompetent, there is a more prolonged "swooooosh" of blood as it regurgitates back down though the incompetent valve.

This can be repeated at any level along the course of the superficial venous systems to assess for perforator incompetence.

TO COMPLETE:

You may mention to the examiner that you would consider assessing the patient's peripheral circulation by feeling for all peripheral pulses and evaluate the neurological status of the limb.

Say you would examine the patient's abdomen for masses and perform a per rectal examination if the history is suggestive of intra-abdominal or pelvic pathology contributing to the varicosities.

You may also wish to consider formal assessment of the peripheral arterial circulation and auscultate the vein for bruits which may represent an arteriovenous fistula. Also check the patient's peripheral neurological status as venous ulcers may be confused with arterial or neuropathic ulcers.

5. Thank the patient

Kean J, Stephen C, Hughes J, Enoch S. Focused Clinical Examination for
MRCS Finals (OSCE). Doctors Academy Publications

BE PREPARED TO ANSWER QUESTIONS ON:

- Anatomical course of long and short saphenous veins and their perforators

- Aetiology, investigations and treatment options of varicose veins

- Complications of varicose vein surgery and post operative instructions

- Investigation and management of venous ulcers

- Deep vein thrombosis and prophylaxis.

Kean J, Stephen C, Hughes J, Enoch S. Focused Clinical Examination for
MRCS Finals (OSCE). Doctors Academy Publications

INDEX

Kean J, Stephen C, Hughes J, Enoch S. Focused Clinical Examination for MRCS Finals (OSCE). Doctors Academy Publications

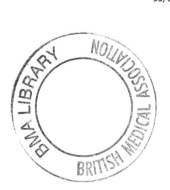
Kean J, Stephen C, Hughes J, Enoch S. Focused Clinical Examination for
MRCS Finals (OSCE). Doctors Academy Publications